HCG DIET

Comprehensive Guide On Food
And Quick Way To Lose Weight.

Walter L. Kelley

Table of Contents

INTRODUCTION

The hormone known as human chorionic gonadotropin (HCG) is produced in both males and females. It is delivered by the placenta in pregnant ladies and is utilized as a marker in pregnancy tests. HCG is also utilized in various medical treatments.

The alpha and beta subunits of the glycoprotein hormone HCG make up the hormone. Other hormones like luteinizing hormone (LH), thyroid-stimulating hormone (TSH), and follicle-stimulating hormone (FSH) share similarities in the alpha subunit. Pregnancy tests use the beta subunit, which is unique to HCG and is used to determine pregnancy. During the first few weeks of pregnancy, HCG levels rise rapidly and reach their maximum around 10 to 12 weeks.

HCG has many uses in medicine. By stimulating ovulation, HCG is used to treat infertility in women. In men, HCG is utilized to increment testosterone creation and treat hypogonadism. HCG is additionally utilized in the therapy of particular kinds of malignant growth, as testicular disease, by forestalling the breakdown of solid cells. By increasing metabolism and decreasing hunger, HCG can also aid in weight loss. HCG, on the other hand, is not approved by the FDA for weight loss and should only be used under the guidance of a medical professional.

CHAPTER1

The history of HCG diet

In recent years, the HCG diet has become increasingly popular as a weight loss plan. Human chorionic gonadotropin, or HCG for short, is a hormone that the placenta makes during pregnancy. A low-calorie diet and daily doses of this hormone are part of the HCG diet. The diet aims to lose weight quickly and effectively without feeling deprived or hungry.

The HCG diet commonly includes a severe calorie admission of just 500-800 calories each day. This is far underneath the normal everyday calorie consumption suggested for most grown-ups. It is thought that the HCG hormone aids in the suppression of hunger and cravings, making it simpler to adhere to the low-calorie diet. The diet typically consists of three phases: stacking, weight reduction, and support. During the stacking stage, which goes on for two days, the singular eats unhealthy food varieties to develop fat stores. The weight reduction stage follows and goes on for three to about a month and a half, during which time the individual consumes an exceptionally low-calorie diet and takes day to day HCG infusions or drops. In order to prevent weight gain, the maintenance phase involves gradually increasing calorie intake and avoiding sugar and starches.

Despite the fact that the HCG diet can help people lose weight, there are risks and debate surrounding it. Experts argue that the weight loss is primarily due to the low calorie intake rather than the HCG hormone, raising questions about the diet's safety and effectiveness. Others warn that people with certain medical conditions or a history of disordered eating may be at risk from the very low-calorie diet. Before beginning any weight loss program, including the HCG diet, it is important to talk to a doctor. The HCG diet is a popular weight loss plan that has gotten a lot of attention in recent years. Human chorionic gonadotropin (HCG) is a hormone that the placenta naturally produces during pregnancy. The HCG diet is based on the idea that this hormone can suppress appetite and speed up metabolism, which can help people lose weight. The diet involves eating very few calories and taking HCG injections or supplements.

The human chorionic gonadotropin (HCG) diet works by tricking the body into thinking it is pregnant, causing it to use stored fat as energy. Because of this, the diet calls for a very low calorie intake, somewhere between 500 and 800 calories per day. The HCG chemical assists with smothering craving and lessen hunger, making it more straightforward to adhere to this prohibitive eating routine. Additionally, it is thought that the hormone speeds up metabolism, which may enable the body to burn more calories even when it is at rest.

Pundits of the HCG diet contend that the weight reduction isn't manageable and that the eating regimen can be perilous because of the very low calorie consumption. However, proponents of the HCG diet assert that it can be an efficient strategy for quick weight loss and overall health improvement. It is essential to keep in mind that the HCG diet should only be followed under the supervision of a medical professional because it may cause adverse effects and not be suitable for all people. In general, the HCG diet is an interesting way to lose weight that people who want to try something new should look into.

During pregnancy, a hormone known as HCG (human chorionic gonadotropin) is produced. It has been used for fertility treatments, but more and more people are using it to help them lose weight. The HCG diet entails daily HCG injections and a strict low-calorie diet. The diet's proponents assert that it can result in significant weight loss, particularly in stubborn areas such as the thighs and stomach. However, just like with any weight loss program, there are pros and cons to keep in mind.

CHAPTER2

The advantages of HCG diet

The HCG diet's ability to accelerate weight loss is one of its main advantages. It is thought that the hormone helps reduce appetite and speeds up the breakdown of stored fat. The diet's proponents also assert that it can assist in resetting the metabolism and encourage long-term weight loss. While on the diet, some also report having more energy and feeling better overall.

The HCG diet, on the other hand, comes with some risks as well.

Nutrient deficiencies and other health issues may result from the strict calorie restriction. In addition, the injections themselves may result in side effects such as irritability, fatigue, and headaches. It is also difficult to determine the diet's safety and efficacy over time due to the lack of research on its long-term effects.

In general, the HCG diet may provide some advantages in terms of rapid weight loss; however, before beginning any new weight loss program, it is essential to take into account the potential risks and speak with a medical professional. Most people think that the safest and most effective way to lose weight is to take a balanced, long-term strategy that includes a healthy diet and regular exercise.

During pregnancy, the placenta makes a hormone called human chorionic gonadotropin (HCG). In addition, it helps people lose weight and has become increasingly popular in recent years. HCG assists in diminishing hunger and advancing fat misfortune from obstinate regions with preferring the mid-region, hips, and thighs. With a low-calorie diet and HCG injections or drops, it is thought that one can quickly lose weight.

CHAPTER3

Tips for HCG diet Conventions

On the off chance that you are wanting to follow the HCG diet, there are a couple of tips that can assist you with accomplishing your weight reduction objectives effectively. Ensure you, first and foremost, counsel a medical care proficient prior to beginning the eating regimen. They are able to look at your health and figure out if the diet is right for you. Second, strictly adhering to the diet plan is essential. This requires adhering to the permitted food list and calorie requirements. Your weight loss progress may be slowed down if you cheat on your diet. Ultimately, it is prescribed to integrate light activity like strolling or yoga into your daily practice. Exercise is good for your health and helps you burn calories.

In conclusion, dieting with HCG can be a quick and effective way to lose weight. However, before beginning, it is essential to seek medical advice and strictly adhere to the diet plan. It can also help you reach your weight loss goals to include some light exercise in your daily routine. With the right methodology, HCG counting calories can be a fruitful weight reduction venture

The HCG Diet Conventions are a health improvement plan with severe rules and conventions. A strict diet and daily injections of the HCG hormone, which is made during pregnancy, make up the program. Rapid weight loss is made possible by the HCG hormone's ability to reduce hunger and speed up metabolism. Due to their efficiency and quick results, the protocols have gained popularity over time.

In the 1950s, Dr. Albert Simons introduced the HCG Diet Protocols for the first time. He discovered that a low-calorie diet and the hormone HCG can help people lose weight quickly. At first, the program was intended for people who were severely overweight or obese. However, in recent years, it has emerged as a well-liked program for those wishing to shed a few pounds.

The HCG Diet Conventions have severe rules and conventions that should be observed to accomplish the ideal outcomes. A specific list of permitted foods, portion sizes, and calorie limits are included in the program. The timing and procedure for giving the HCG injections are also covered in the guidelines. To ensure the program's effectiveness and achieve the desired outcomes, it is essential to follow the protocols.

The HCG Diet Conventions is a weight reduction routine that consolidates a low-calorie diet with ordinary dosages of the chemical human chorionic gonadotropin (HCG). The eating regimen is partitioned into four stages, each with its own arrangement of rules and limitations. In stage 1, otherwise called the Stacking Stage, weight watchers are permitted to eat fatty food sources for two days while taking HCG supplements.

During the Stacking Stage, weight watchers are permitted to eat anything they desire, particularly high-fat food varieties. This is due to the fact that the phase's goal is to fill the body with calories and store fat in anticipation of the next phase, which restricts calories. Burgers, fries, pizza, ice cream, and other high-calorie foods are allowed during this phase. However, starchy and sugary foods, for example, should be avoided because they can compromise HCG's effectiveness.

CHAPTER 4

The Phases of HCG of diet

The HCG Diet Protocols' success depends on the Loading Phase, even though it may seem counterintuitive to eat high-calorie foods. By devouring fatty food sources for two days, the body is prepared to enter the calorie-limited stage, during which weight watchers will eat just 500-800 calories each day. The individuals who skip or hurry through the Stacking Stage are probably going to encounter craving and shortcoming during the calorie-confined stage, prompting a more serious gamble of abandoning the eating routine. To ensure success in the subsequent phases, it is crucial to adhere to the Loading Phase's guidelines.

The HCG diet is a way to lose weight that uses drops or injections of the hormone human chorionic gonadotropin (HCG). Each of the four phases of the diet has its own set of guidelines and restrictions. The low-calorie diet phase of the HCG diet typically lasts between 21 and 40 days. Participants are required to follow a very low-calorie diet (VLCD) of 500 to 800 calories per day during this phase.

During phase 2 of the HCG diet, very specific and limited foods are allowed. Lean proteins like chicken, fish, and lean beef, as well as vegetables like spinach, lettuce, and tomatoes, make up the majority of the diet. Natural products like apples, grapefruits, and strawberries are additionally permitted, however in exceptionally restricted amounts. Notwithstanding these food varieties, members may likewise eat specific flavors and sauces, like salt, pepper, mustard, and vinegar.

Then again, there are likewise various food varieties that are confined or disallowed during stage 2 of the HCG diet. Sugar, bread, pasta, and rice, as well as fatty meats, dairy, and oils, are examples of foods with a lot of calories. Chips, crackers, and other snack foods that are processed are also prohibited. The HCG diet can only be successful if these food restrictions are strictly adhered to. Any deviation from the prescribed diet could cause weight gain or other negative effects.

The human chorionic gonadotropin (HCG) hormone is used in conjunction with a low-calorie diet in the popular HCG diet for weight loss. The program is partitioned into various stages, each with its own arrangement of rules and rules. The stabilization phase, also known as phase 3, of the HCG diet is one of its most crucial phases.

The primary goal of the stabilization phase is to keep the weight loss from the previous phases of the program. This stage goes on for quite a long time, and during this time, there are sure food varieties that are permitted and others that are confined. The primary objective is to gradually increase calorie intake while avoiding foods that can cause weight gain.

A portion of the food sources that are permitted during the adjustment period of the HCG diet incorporate lean proteins like chicken, fish, and turkey, as well as organic products, vegetables, and solid fats like avocados and nuts. However, certain foods, such as sugar, processed foods, and starchy vegetables like corn and potatoes, must be avoided during this time. Additionally, alcohol should be avoided during this phase because it can hinder efforts to maintain weight.

All in all, the adjustment period of the HCG diet is basic for keeping up with the weight reduction accomplished during the past periods of the program. During this stage, there are sure food sources that are permitted and others that are confined, with the objective of continuously expanding calorie consumption while keeping away from weight gain. Individuals can successfully transition to a long-term, healthy lifestyle by adhering to the guidelines and consuming healthy foods.

The HCG Diet Protocol is a program for losing weight that has recently gained a lot of popularity. It is intended to assist people with getting more fit rapidly and successfully by observing severe dietary rules and taking HCG chemical enhancements. The maintenance phase, also known as phase 4, is one of this diet plan's most important phases. People need to be careful about the foods they eat and stick to certain dietary restrictions during this phase.

The HCG Diet Protocol's maintenance phase is important because it helps people stabilize their weight loss and keep it off. During this stage, people are urged to eat a solid, adjusted diet comprising of entire food sources, lean proteins, and complex starches. Sugar, starches, and processed foods are among the foods that are restricted during this phase. These foods must not be eaten because they can make you gain weight and mess up the body's natural metabolism.

Those who are in the maintenance phase of the HCG Diet Protocol are not only subjected to dietary restrictions, but they are also encouraged to lead active lifestyles. Maintaining weight loss and enhancing one's overall health and well-being are both aided by regular exercise and physical activity. During this phase, regular weight monitoring is also essential to ensuring that weight stays within a healthy range. The HCG Diet Protocol can help individuals maintain their weight loss and achieve long-term success if they adhere to these guidelines and restrictions.

A well-liked diet plan called the HCG Diet Food Guide makes use of a hormone called human chorionic gonadotropin (HCG). This chemical is normally created by ladies during pregnancy and is accepted to assist with managing digestion and consume fat. The diet entails daily injections or drops of HCG and a very low calorie intake, typically between 500 and 800 calories per day. The diet aims to assist individuals in losing weight quickly and effectively.

. The diet has been reported to have helped many people lose up to one pound per day. People who have previously struggled with weight loss may find this very motivating. Additionally, the diet promises to aid in weight loss while preserving muscle mass, which is essential for sustaining a healthy metabolism.

The possibility of sustained weight loss is yet another advantage of the HCG Diet. The diet aims to speed up metabolism and encourage healthier eating habits. People may be able to keep their weight loss over time if they follow the diet and incorporate healthy habits into their daily lives. Furthermore, the eating routine might assist with peopling break undesirable examples of eating and foster a superior relationship with food.

In general, the HCG Diet Food Guide can be an efficient and quick way to lose weight. But before you start the diet, it's important to talk to a doctor or other medical professional to make sure it's safe for you. Furthermore, it is critical to follow the eating regimen intently and integrate sound propensities into your everyday daily practice to accomplish long haul weight reduction achievement.

The popular HCG Diet Food Guide is a weight loss plan that requires injections of Human Chorionic Gonadotropin (HCG) hormone and strict adherence to a low-calorie diet. The low-calorie diet helps the body burn off stored fat, and the HCG hormone is thought to suppress appetite and promote fat burning. There are some foods that can be eaten while following the HCG Diet, while others are not. In this article, we will examine the permitted food varieties on the HCG Diet.

CHAPTER5

Foods to follow in HCG diet
And avoid

There is a limited amount of food that can be consumed on the HCG Diet that is low in calories, high in protein, and low in sugar, fat, carbohydrates, and other sugars. Lean proteins like chicken breast, beef, fish, and shellfish are included in these foods. Also permitted are vegetables like asparagus, spinach, lettuce, tomatoes, and cucumbers. Likewise, natural products like apples, oranges, and strawberries can be consumed in modest quantities.

When following the HCG Diet, portion control is one of the most important things to keep in mind. The HCG Diet's permitted foods must be consumed in specific quantities and at specific times throughout the day. For instance, a breakfast may consist of one serving of protein, one serving of fruit, and black coffee or tea. One serving of fruit, one serving of vegetables, and one serving of protein may be included in your lunch. Supper might comprise of one protein serving, one vegetable serving, and one organic product serving. Snacks are not permitted on the HCG Diet.

All in all, the HCG Diet Food Guide is a weight reduction plan that requires a severe adherence to a low-calorie diet and the utilization of HCG chemical infusions. Permitted food sources on the HCG Diet incorporate lean proteins, vegetables, and organic products. When following the HCG Diet, portion control is essential because allowed foods must be consumed in specific amounts and at specific times throughout the day. If you want to lose weight quickly, the HCG Diet is a good option. However, you should only follow it with the help of a medical professional.

The HCG diet is a get-healthy plan that includes taking human chorionic gonadotropin, a chemical created during pregnancy, and following a severe low-calorie diet. The HCG diet aims to assist individuals in losing weight quickly and effectively. However, the food guide must be strictly followed in order to maximize the benefits of this diet. A list of foods that can and cannot be eaten while following the HCG diet is included in the food guide.

The list of foods to avoid is one of the most crucial aspects of the HCG diet food guide. Foods with a lot of calories, sugar, and fat are on this list. The justification for staying away from these food varieties is that they can obstruct the hormonal equilibrium that the HCG chemical makes in the body. Sugar, processed foods, dairy products, grains, and other foods should not be eaten on the HCG diet. These foods might spike insulin, which could make you gain weight.

One more food class to stay away from on the HCG diet is high-fat food sources. Consuming high-fat foods can disrupt the HCG hormone's ability to burn fat, resulting in weight gain rather than loss. Butter, oils, fatty meats, cheese, and other foods in this category should be avoided. If consumed while following the HCG diet, these high-calorie foods may cause weight gain.

In conclusion, one must adhere to the HCG diet food guide in order to achieve maximum weight loss results. Sugar, processed foods, dairy products, grains, high-fat foods, butter, oils, fatty meats, and cheese are all things you should avoid on the HCG diet. One can achieve the desired weight loss outcomes by avoiding these foods and maintaining the hormonal equilibrium that the HCG hormone creates in the body. The HCG diet is an effective weight loss plan that has recently gained popularity. It is a low-calorie diet that includes taking HCG supplements, either through infusions or drops, while devouring a particular arrangement of food varieties. Lean proteins and vegetables are emphasized in the HCG diet food guide, and carbohydrate and fat intake are limited.

With regards to feast anticipating the HCG diet, it is crucial for adhere to the supported food list. Lean meats like chicken breast, shrimp, and lean beef are on this list, as are vegetables like asparagus, spinach, and tomatoes. Fruits are permitted, but due to their high sugar content, they should be consumed in moderation. The HCG diet food guide likewise suggests restricting the admission of bland starches and fats, like bread and butter.

A breakfast of two egg whites scrambled with spinach and tomatoes or a cup of Greek yogurt with a small handful of berries could be included in a sample HCG diet meal plan. Grilled chicken breast with steamed asparagus could be served for lunch, and grilled shrimp with a side salad of mixed greens and cherry tomatoes could be served for dinner. A handful of almonds or an apple with a tablespoon of almond butter are examples of snacks that can be consumed in between meals. Following a feast plan like this can assist people on the HCG with counting calories accomplish their weight reduction objectives while as yet consuming nutritious and fulfilling dinners.

In conclusion, the HCG diet is a low-calorie weight loss plan that places an emphasis on vegetables and lean proteins and restricts carbs and fats. It is essential for success on the HCG diet to adhere to the food guide; individuals should eat foods that are permitted while avoiding those that are not. Lean proteins like grilled chicken breast or shrimp and steamed vegetables or a side salad may be included in a sample HCG diet meal plan. A handful of almonds or an apple with almond butter are examples of snacks that can be consumed in the time between meals. People on the

HCG diet can achieve their weight loss goals while still eating nutritious and filling meals by following a meal plan like this.

Due to its promising weight loss results, the HCG diet has gained a lot of popularity in recent years. A low-calorie diet and supplements of human chorionic gonadotropin (HCG) are required. However, in order to get the most out of this diet, certain success strategies must be followed. To begin, adhering to the recommended food guide is essential to consuming only permitted foods. Lean proteins, vegetables, fruits, and a small amount of carbohydrates are included in this guide. For best results, you should also avoid alcohol, sugary drinks, and processed foods.

CHAPTER 6

Meal planning in the HCG diet

Planning your meals in advance is yet another important tip for achieving success on the HCG diet. You'll be able to stay on track and avoid straying from the diet plan thanks to this. Feast arranging likewise guarantees that you have every one of the essential elements for your dinners, which recoveries time and disposes of the requirement for somewhat late outings to the supermarket. In addition, it is suggested that you cook your meals at home rather than eating out because doing so gives you complete control over the ingredients and methods of cooking.

Last but not least, success on the HCG diet depends on staying hydrated. Not only does drinking a lot of water help flush out toxins from your body, but it also helps you feel less hungry and less hungry-for-food. To keep your body hydrated, it is recommended that you drink at least 2 liters of water each day. You can likewise polish off different liquids like home grown teas or weakened natural product juices. However, as they can hinder the success of the diet, it is essential to stay away from drinks that contain sugar or artificial sweeteners. You can succeed on the HCG diet and achieve your weight loss goals in a healthy and long-lasting manner if you follow these guidelines.

The HCG diet is a get-healthy plan that includes the utilization of the chemical human chorionic gonadotropin (HCG), which is created during pregnancy. The strict 500-calorie daily diet and daily injections of HCG are part of this diet. The HCG diet is expected to help you lose a lot of weight, usually between 1 and 2 pounds per day. However, it is essential to keep in mind that the HCG injections were not the only factor in the weight loss. Additionally, the low-calorie diet is a significant contributor to weight loss.

The HCG diet aims to lose fat while maintaining muscle mass. The chemical is accepted to assist with stifling craving and increment digestion, which prompts fast weight reduction. Furthermore, it's remembered to assist with reallocating fat from pain points like the hips, thighs, and stomach. The HCG diet works for many people who try it and lose a lot of weight quickly. But it's important to remember that the

HCG diet doesn't work long-term. It is common for people to regain the weight they lost after stopping the diet.

While the HCG diet might prompt quick weight reduction, it's not without gambles. Headaches, fatigue, irritability, dizziness, and other side effects of the low-calorie diet are among the potential side effects. A number of health risks, including blood clots, depression, and ovarian hyperstimulation syndrome (OHSS), have also been linked to the use of HCG injections. OHSS is a condition where the ovaries become enlarged and excruciating. It has the potential to be fatal in severe cases. When considering the HCG diet, it is essential to weigh the potential benefits and risks.

The HCG diet is a get-healthy plan that includes taking a chemical called human chorionic gonadotropin (HCG) alongside a low-calorie diet. While advocates of the HCG diet guarantee that it can assist individuals with getting more fit rapidly and actually, there are additionally possible dangers and secondary effects that ought to be viewed as prior to beginning this eating routine.

One of the super possible dangers of the HCG diet is that it can prompt supplement inadequacies. It may be challenging to obtain all of the vitamins and minerals your body needs to function properly because the diet involves severely restricting calories. Fatigue, weakness, and other health issues may result from this. Additionally, side effects associated with the HCG hormone itself include nausea, dizziness, and headaches.

The HCG diet has the potential to cause muscle loss, which is yet another potential drawback. Your body will begin to burn both muscle and fat for energy if you cut back on calories. During this process, the HCG hormone is thought to help preserve muscle mass. It's possible that if you don't take the hormone, you'll lose more muscle than fat, which could be bad for your health as a whole.

By and large, while the HCG diet might be compelling for certain individuals, gauging the likely dangers and aftereffects prior to beginning this program is significant. If you decide to try the HCG diet, you should talk to your doctor first to make sure it is safe for you and to keep a close eye on your health during the process. Furthermore, it's vital to ensure that you're getting each of the supplements that your body needs to work appropriately, even while on a low-calorie diet.

Taking a hormone called human chorionic gonadotropin (HCG) in conjunction with a very low-calorie diet is a popular weight loss strategy. The eating routine professes to assist individuals with getting thinner quickly, for certain defenders guaranteeing that individuals can lose as much as a pound a day. This diet might work for some people, but it also comes with significant risks that people should be aware of. Gallstone formation, electrolyte imbalances, and nutritional deficiencies are some of the risks.

However, there are measures that can be taken to lessen the risks of the HCG diet. Before beginning the diet, the first step is to talk to a doctor. Because the HCG hormone can interact with some medications, this is especially important for people who have underlying health conditions or who take medications. While on a diet, people should also make sure they are getting enough nutrients. This can be accomplished by taking a multivitamin or by integrating supplement rich food varieties into the eating routine.

The strict adherence to the diet plan is yet another way to reduce the risks associated with the HCG diet. The HCG diet typically restricts calories to 500-800 per day, which is significantly less than the daily allowance for most people. This has the potential to starve the body, which can result in a variety of health issues. Protein and fiber, which can help people feel full and provide the body with the nutrients it needs to function properly, should be included in people's diets to lower their risk of these issues.

Overall, the HCG diet can be a quick and effective way to lose weight, but there are some downsides. Before beginning the diet, individuals should consult a physician, ensure that they are consuming sufficient nutrients, and adhere strictly to the plan. People can achieve the results they want without jeopardizing their health by following these steps

Although the HCG diet has been around for a few decades, it has recently received a lot of attention due to its potential for rapid weight loss. However, due to its potential risks, the HCG diet has also received significant criticism from the medical community. Despite this, people continue to try the HCG diet, so it's important to look more closely at its benefits and drawbacks.

The HCG diet has been demonstrated to result in rapid weight loss. This is primarily attributable to the diet's low calorie intake and HCG injections. The HCG chemical should stifle craving and increment digestion, which can, thus, lead to weight reduction. However, the individual's weight loss is not long-lasting, and once they return to their normal diet, it usually comes back.

Then again, the possible dangers of the HCG diet can't be disregarded. Right off the bat, the HCG chemical isn't FDA endorsed for weight reduction. Furthermore, the low-calorie admission of the eating routine can prompt hunger and other medical conditions. Additionally, the HCG diet has the potential to cause adverse effects such as fatigue, mood swings, headaches, and even blood clots. Before beginning the HCG diet, individuals should speak with their doctors about the potential side effects.

All in all, the HCG diet can create quick weight reduction, however the outcomes are not economical. Before beginning the HCG diet, individuals should take into account the significant risks. Medical professionals do not recommend the HCG diet, so before beginning any weight loss program, people should talk to their doctor. In the end, the best strategy for long-term weight loss and overall health is a healthy weight loss plan that includes a balanced diet and regular exercise.

THE END